# Your Delicious In
# Vegetaria

## A Full Collection of Vegetarian Recipes to Begin Your Diet Program and Improve Your Health

America Best Recipes

Table of Contents

**Breakfast**

**Whole Wheat Chapatti**

Servings: 8 servings Preparation Time: 10 mins Cooking Time: 10 mins

Ingredients:

2½ cups whole wheat flour

¾ tsp.

salt

1 cup water

Directions:

In a medium-sized bowl, mix the flour and salt and then stir in water to form a soft, pliable dough. Scrape the dough out onto a lightly floured and clean work surface. Using your hands, knead several times to improve the dough's elasticity and smoothness. Divide the dough into 8 equal portions and roll each into a smooth ball. Roll each ball into a fragile circle. Heat a griddle pan over a medium-high heat. Do not add any oil. Cook each dough round on the pan until the dough begins to bubbles and blister, about 2 minutes. Flip over and cook until lightly brown on the other side. Serve immediately.

## Hot Pink Smoothie

Preparation time: 5 minutes Cooking time: 0 minute

Servings: 1

Ingredients:

1 clementine, peeled, segmented

1/2 frozen banana

1 small beet, peeled, chopped

1/8 teaspoon sea salt

1/2 cup raspberries

1 tablespoon chia seeds

1/4 teaspoon vanilla extract, unsweetened

2 tablespoons almond butter

1 cup almond milk, unsweetened


Directions:

Place all the ingredients in the order in a food processor or blender and then pulse for 2 to 3 minutes at high speed until smooth. Pour the smoothie into a glass and then serve.

## Chocolate Oat Smoothie

Preparation time: 5 minutes Cooking time: 0 minute

Servings: 1

Ingredients:

¼ cup rolled oats

1 ½ tablespoon cocoa powder, unsweetened

1 teaspoon flax seeds

1 large frozen banana

1/8 teaspoon sea salt

1/8  teaspoon cinnamon

¼ teaspoon vanilla extract, unsweetened

2 tablespoons almond butter

1 cup coconut milk, unsweetened


Directions:

Place all the ingredients in the ordr in a food processor or blender and then pulse for 2 to 3 minutes at high speed until smooth. Pour the smoothie into a glass and then serve.

## Wild Ginger Green Smoothie

Preparation time: 5 minutes Cooking time: 0 minute

Servings: 1

Ingredients:

1/2 cup pineapple chunks, frozen

1/2 cup chopped kale

1/2 frozen banana

1 tablespoon lime juice

2 inches ginger, peeled, chopped

1/2 cup coconut milk, unsweetened

1/2 cup coconut water

Directions:

Place all the ingredients in the order in a food processor or blender and then pulse for 2 to 3 minutes at high speed until smooth. Pour the smoothie into a glass and then serve.

## Double Chocolate Hazelnut Espresso Shake

Preparation time: 5 minutes Cooking time: 0 minute

Servings: 1

Ingredients:

1 frozen banana, sliced

1/4 cup roasted hazelnuts

4 Medjool dates, pitted, soaked

2 tablespoons cacao nibs, unsweetened

1 1/2 tablespoons cacao powder, unsweetened

1/8 teaspoon sea salt

1 teaspoon vanilla extract, unsweetened

1 cup almond milk, unsweetened

1/2 cup ice

4 ounces espresso, chilled

Directions:

Place all the ingredients in the order in a food processor or blender and then pulse for 2 to 3 minutes at high speed until smooth. Pour the smoothie into a glass and then serve.

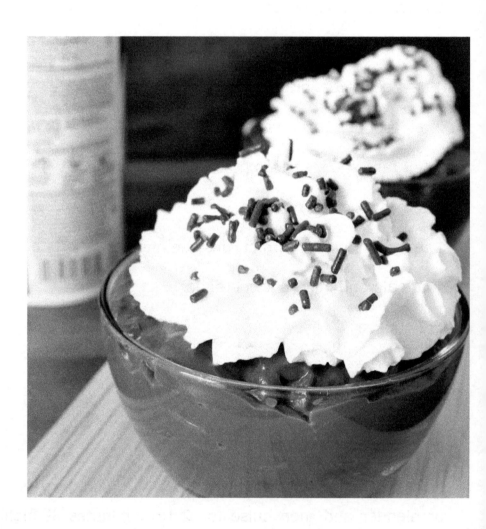

## Cauliflower Casserole

Prep time: 6 min Cooking Time: 20 min Serve: 2

Ingredients

1 cup tofu

1 cup chopped cauliflower

½ cup shredded goat cheese

2 eggs, lightly beaten

2 tablespoons almond flour

2 teaspoons coconut oil

1 1/2 tablespoons finely chopped onion

1/8 teaspoon salt

Additional shredded goat cheese, optional


Instructions

In an Instant Pot, press Sauté and add coconut oil when hot. Add the onion, sauté until the onion are tender, about 5 minutes.

Add the all ingredients in the Instant Pot and lock lid and set pressure release valve to Sealing. Press Manual or Pressure Cooker; cook at High Pressure 15 minutes.

When cooking is complete, use Natural-release for 10 minutes, then release remaining pressure.

Serve and enjoy.

Nutrition Facts

Calories 247, Total Fat 17.6g, Saturated Fat 8.2g, Cholesterol 171mg, Sodium 264mg, Total Carbohydrate 6.1g, Dietary Fiber 2.7g, Total Sugars 2.7g, Protein 19.5g

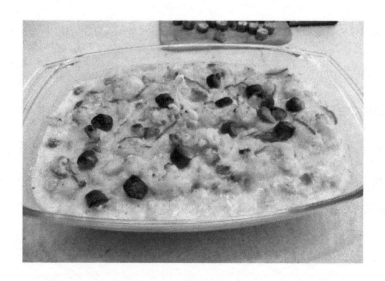

## Chocolate Millet

Prep time: 05 min Cooking Time: 6 ½ hours Serve: 2

Ingredients

1 cup millet

3 cups water

½ cup almond milk

1 tablespoon cocoa powder

¼ teaspoon cinnamon

¼ teaspoon vanilla

½ cup blueberry

Chocolate chips and dried fruit for topping

Instructions

Add all ingredients to Instant Pot and stir. Ensure the lid is set to "Sealing" and set Slow Cook function to cook for 6 ½ hours.

Spoon into bowls and top with a sprinkle of chocolate chips and blueberry.

Nutrition Facts

Calories 545, Total Fat 19g, Saturated Fat 13.6g, Cholesterol 0mg, Sodium 26mg, Total Carbohydrate

83.2g, Dietary Fiber 11.7g, Total Sugars 5.7g, Protein 13.2g

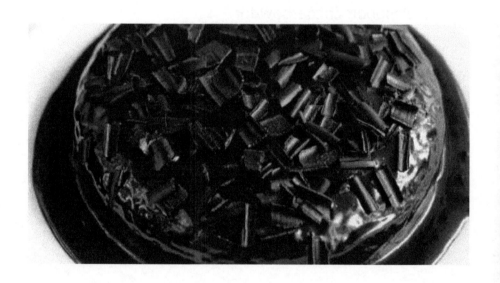

## Breakfast Hash

Prep time: 05 min Cooking Time: 05 min Serve: 2

Ingredients

1 tablespoon coconut oil

2 small sweet potatoes, peeled if desired

2 eggs

1/4 cup water

1 cup shredded parmesan cheese

Instructions

Set the Instant Pot to "Sauté" and add a thin layer of coconut oil to the bottom of the pan. While the Instant Pot is heating, finely shred the sweet potatoes in a food processor. Squeeze out any excess moisture then add the shredded sweet potatoes to the hot oil. Let the sweet potatoes brown in the hot oil without stirring.

Meanwhile, beat the eggs and set aside.

Once the sweet potatoes have browned on the bottom, break them up with a wooden spoon. Add the water, eggs, parmesan cheese, Stir gently.

Lock the cover on the Instant Pot and let cook for 1 minute then use the Quick-release method to release the steam.

Serve the breakfast hash immediately.

Nutrition Facts

Calories 344, Total Fat 14.4g, Saturated Fat 9.3g, Cholesterol 174mg, Sodium 206mg, Total Carbohydrate 42.7g, Dietary Fiber 6.2g, Total Sugars 1.1g, Protein 12.3g

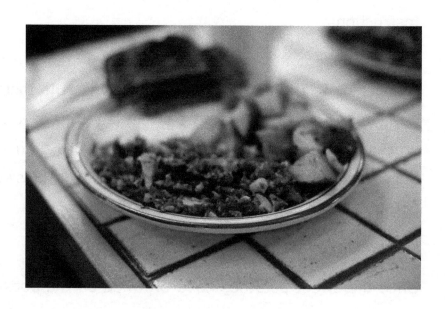

## Omelette Quiche

Prep time: 05 min Cooking Time: 30 min Serve: 2

Ingredients

2 large eggs (beaten)

⅛ teaspoon salt and pepper

½ cup Jalapeño pepper (diced)

1 green onion

¼ cup coconut milk

2 tablespoons cheddar cheese (shredded)

1½ cups of water

½ tablespoon butter/cooking oil


Instructions

Place the metal trivet or long handled trivet in the bottom of your Instant Pot and add 1½ cups of water.

Butter or spray your dish with cooking oil.

In a large mixing bowl whisk together the eggs, milk, salt and pepper. Add diced Jalapeño peppers, green onion slices, and cheese to your prepared plate, then mix well.

Pour egg mixture over to top of the vegetables and stir to combine.

Loosely cover the dish with aluminium foil or silicone lid cover. Use either an aluminium foil sling or the long handled trivet to place the dish in the Instant Pot liner.

Lock lid in place and select Manual. Press the Pressure Cooker button and set the cook time for 30 minutes at High Pressure. Allow it to count up to 10 minutes, hit [Cancel] to turn off, then use a quick pressure release.

Remove the foil. If desired, sprinkle the top of the western quiche with additional cheese. Serve immediately .


Nutrition Facts

Calories112, Total Fat 7.4g, Saturated Fat 3g,Cholesterol 193mg ,Sodium 503mg, Total Carbohydrate 3.3g, Dietary Fiber 0.6g, , Total Sugars 2.1g, Protein 8.5g

# French Toast

Prep time: 05 min Cooking Time: 25 min Serve: 2

Ingredients

1 cup almond milk

1 egg

1 teaspoon honey

1/2 teaspoon almond extract

1/4 teaspoon nutmeg

1/8 cup fresh strawberry

2 thick slices French bread cut into 2-inch pieces

Cooking spray

3/4 cup water

Directions

In a bowl, put together milk, egg, honey, almond extract, and nutmeg until well blended.

Fold in the strawberry and bread pieces until well coated.

Spray the baking dish with cooking spray and pour the bread mixture into the dish.

Place the steam rack into the Instant Pot inner pot and add 3/4 cup water. Carefully lower the baking dish onto the steam rack.

Lock lid, ensuring the valve is turned to the Sealing position.

Press the Pressure Cooker button and set the time to 25 minutes.

Nutrition Facts

Calories 423, Total Fat 31.8g, Saturated Fat 26.3g, Cholesterol 82mg, Sodium 257mg, Total Carbohydrate 29.3g, Dietary Fiber 3.7g , Total Sugars 9g, Protein 9.4g

**Lunch**
**Low Carb Taco Shells**

Soft Low carb spinach taco shells makes a delicious replacement to regular tacos.

Prep Time: 10 mins Cook Time: 15 mins Total Time: 25 mins

Ingredients

4 oz Fresh Spinach Leaves (100 g)

4 cups Boiling Water

2 Egg

4 tablespoon Almond Flour or oat flour

1/2 cup Grated Cheese

1/4 teaspoon Garlic powder - optional

1/4 teaspoon salt - optional

Instructions

Preheat oven to 390 F (200 C).

Place the fresh spinach leaves into a large mixing bowl.

Cover the spinach leaves with 4 cups of boiling water. Cover. Set aside 2 minutes.

In another bowl add ice cubes, about 1 cup.

Using tongs remove the cooked spinach leaves from the mixing bowl and place them into the bowl filled with ice cubes. Stir the leaves into the ice cubes for few seconds to cool down.

Squeeze the spinach leaves with your hands to remove all the water. It will form a compact spinach 'ball.'

Pat dry the spinach between layers of absorbent paper to ensure that the cooked spinach are fully dry.

Finely chopped the cooked spinach on a chopping board.

Place them into a large mixing bowl and combine with grated cheese, eggs and almond meal, garlic powder and salt until it forms a sort of batter.

Scoop out the batter onto a baking tray covered with parchment paper. I recommend to spray some olive oil on the parchment paper too to avoid the shells to stick to the paper ! I used a mechanical ice cream scoop maker to scoop out the batter into 4 equal amount of taco shell batter.

Use your fingers to flatten each scoop of taco batter into a evenly flat thin circle that looks like a taco.

Bake at 390 F (200 C) for 15 minutes or until it is golden and crispy on sides. Depending on oven and thickness of your tacos you may have to reduce to 350 F (180C). Simply watch the color and texture while baking to avoid burning. It is baked when the border are crispy and slighty golden brown.

Cool down on a plate few minutes before eating.

Can be eaten lukewarm or cold with toppings of your choice.

Toppings ideas: lettuce, scramble eggs, tomatoes, avocado and sriracha sauce for a delicious breakfast or grilled vegetables, tofu, chicken. Any of your favorite taco fillings will be delicious in those shells/Cheese: use any hard grated cheese like mozzarella, cheddar, emmental, edam or colby

Freezing: freeze well in airtight container. Make sure the shells don't overlap or it make them difficult to defrost individually. Place a piece of parchment paper between each taco to avoid this problem. Defrost in less than 1 hour at room temperature. Rewarm in sandwich wrap or hot oven 1-2 minutes at 150 C (300f).

Nutrition Info

Amount Per Serving (1 shell) Calories 75

Calories from Fat 50 Fat 5.5g Carbohydrates 2.5g Fiber 1.4g

Sugar 0.5g Protein 4.8g Net Carbs 1.1g

# Avocado Baked Eggs

Prep Time: 10 mins Cook Time: 15 mins Total Time: 25 mins Servings: 2 servings

Ingredients

1 avocado, medium sized 2 eggs

shredded cheddar cheese kosher salt

freshly ground black pepper

Instructions

Preheat oven to 425 degrees.

Slice the avocado in half and remove the pit. With a spoon, carve out enough avocado to make room for the egg.

Place avocado halves onto the backside of muffin pan to stabilize them while cooking.

Crack open an egg into each half of the avocado. Depending on the size of your egg, you may have excess egg white.

Season with salt and pepper.

Sprinkle halves with cheese and place pan in the oven for 13-16 mins depending on the yolk consistency you desire.

Serve immediately, top with Sriracha for a little kick of flavor.

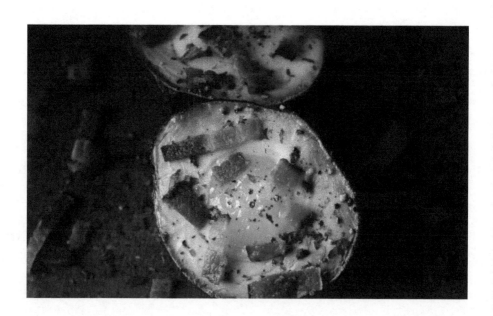

# Cauliflower Crust Grilled Cheese

Makes 2

Ingredients

Cauliflower crust "bread" slices

1 small head cauliflower, cut into small florets (should Servings 3 cups of cauliflower rice)

1 free-range organic egg, lightly beaten

½ cup / 1.7 oz / 50 gr shredded mozzarella cheese

½ teaspoon fine grain sea salt

¼ teaspoon ground black pepper Grilled cheese

Instructions

1      tablespoon butter, room temperature

⅓ cup / 3 oz / 85 gr sharp cheddar cheese, grated/shredded, at room temperature

Cauliflower crust "bread" slices

Preheat oven to 450°F (220°C) and place a rack in the middle. Line a baking sheet with parchment paper and liberally grease it with olive oil. Set aside.

In a food processor rice the cauliflower florets (it should be evenly chopped but not wholly pulverized).

Transfer cauliflower rice (about 3 cups) to a microwave-safe dish and microwave on high for 8 minutes, until cooked.

Place the cauliflower rice in a dishcloth (or tea towel) and twist it to squeeze as much moisture as you can (I usually squeeze out over a cup of liquid). This is very important. The cauliflower rice needs to be dry, otherwise you'll end up with mushy dough, impossible to use as slices of bread.

Transfer the cauliflower rice to a mixing bowl, add egg, mozzarella, salt, pepper and mix well.

Spread cauliflower mixture onto the lined baking sheet and shape into 4 squares.

Place in the oven and bake for about 16 minutes until golden. Remove and let cool 10 minutes before peeling them off the parchment paper (be careful not to break them!)

Assemble cauliflower crust grilled cheese

Heat a pan over medium heat.

Butter one side of each slice of cauliflower crust bread (preferably the top part).

Place one slice of bread in the pan, buttered side down, sprinkle with the cheese and top with the remaining slice of cauliflower crust bread, buttered side up.

Turn the heat down a notch and cook until golden brown, about 2 to 4 minutes.

Gently flip and cook until golden brown on the other side, about 2 to 4 minutes.


Nutrition Info

374 calories 29 grams of fat

8 grams of carbs

23 grams of protein.

# Quick Keto McMuffins

Hands-on 10 minutes Total Time: 10 minutes

Ingredients (makes 2 servings)

Muffins:

1/4 cup almond flour (25 g/ 0.9 oz)

1/4 cup flaxmeal (38 g/ 1.3 oz)

1/4 tsp baking soda

1 large egg, free-range or organic

2 tbsp heavy whipping cream or coconut milk

2 tbsp water

1/4 cup grated cheddar cheese or other Italian hard cheese (28 g/ 1 oz)

pinch of salt

Filling:

2 large eggs

1 tbsp ghee (you can make your own)

1 tbsp butter or 2 tbsp cream cheese for spreading

2 slices cheddar cheese or other hard type cheese (56 g/ 2 oz)

1 tsp Dijon mustard or 2 tsp sugar-free ketchup (you can make your own)

salt and pepper to taste

Optional: 2 cups greens (lettuce, kale, chard, spinach, watercress, etc.)

Optional: 4 slices crisped up bacon or Pancetta

Instructions

Place all the dry ingredients in a small bowl and cmbine well. Quick Keto McMuffins

Add the egg, cream, water and mix well using a fork. Quick Keto McMuffins

Grate the cheese and add it to the mixture. Combine well and place in single-serving ramekins. Quick Keto McMuffins Microwave on high for 60-90 seconds.

Quick Keto McMuffins

Meanwhile, fry the eggs on ghee. I used small pancake molds to create perfect shapes for the muffin. Cook the eggs until the egg white is opaque and the yolks still runny. Season with salt and pepper and take off the heat. Quick Keto McMuffins

Cut the muffins in half and spread some butter on the inside of each of the halves. Quick Keto McMuffins

Top each with slices of cheese, egg and mustard. Optionally, serve with greens (lettuce, spinach, watercress, chard, etc.) and bacon. Quick Keto McMuffins

Enjoy immediately! The muffins (without the filling) can be stored in an airtight container for up to 3 days. You can also freeze them fr up to 3 months.


Nutrition Info

Net carbs3.7 grams Protein25.6 grams Fat54.7 grams Calories627 kcal

# Chile Rellenos Bake

This low-carb vegetarian Chili Rellenos Bake is just as delicious as the Chile Rellenos you get in a restaurant!

Prep Time 20 minutes Cook Time 40 minutes Total Time 1 hour Servings 8 servings

Ingredients

1 27 oz. can roasted and peeled green chiles (see notes)

4 cups grated Four-Cheese Mexican blend cheese

1/2 cup very thinly sliced green onions (optional)

5 eggs

1/2 cup half and half (see notes)

1/2 tsp. ground cumin

1/2 tsp. chile powder

Instructions

Put green chiles in a colander placed in the sink and let drain for about 15 minutes.

While chiles drain, preheat oven to 375F/190C.

Spray glass or crockery casserole dish with non-stick spray or olive oil. (I used a 9" X 13" dish, but anything close to that size will work.)

When chiles are drained, use your thumb to split open each chile, scrape out seeds, and spread chiles out on a paper towel to drain more, pressing down with another towel to get them as dry as you can. (I like to make 2 piles after I do this to get the layers even.)

Make a flat layer of chiles covering the bottom of the dish. (I alternated every other chile facing the opposite way because they're slightly v-shaped.)

Top the layer of chiles with half the grated cheese, then sprinkle on green onions (if using).

Make another layer of flattened chiles, followed by the rest of the cheese.

Put eggs into a bowl and beat well, then add half and half, ground cumin, and chile powder, and stir until well combined. Pour egg mixture over chiles and cheese, taking care to get it evenly distributed. (The egg mixture will not completely cover the casserole.)

Cover dish with foil for the first 15 minutes of baking time, then remove foil and continue to bake until mixture is bubbling and cheese on top is lightly browned, about 40 minutes total baking time.

You can cook it without the foil, but watch it carefully or the top will get too brown. Cooking time without foil will be slightly less.

Serve hot, with sour cream and salsa if desired.

This will keep in the fridge for a few days, and reheats beautifully.

Nutrition Info

Calories: 139 Total Fat: 10g Saturated Fat: 5g

Unsaturated Fat: 4g Cholesterol: 139mg Sodium: 159mg Carbohydrates: 4.8g Sugar: 1

Protein: 9g

# Roasted Lemon Green Beans and Red Potatoes

Ingredients

1 1/2 pounds red potatoes, cut into chunks

2 tablespoons salted butter

12 cloves garlic, thinly sliced

1 tbsp. lemon juice

1 tsp. annatto seeds

2 teaspoons sea salt

1 bunch green beans, trimmed and cut into 1 inch pieces

Directions:

Preheat your oven to 425 degrees F. In a baking pan, combine the first 5 ingredients and 1/2 of the sea salt. Cover with foil. Bake 20 minutes in the oven. Combine the asparagus, oil, and salt. Cover, and cook for about 15 minutes, or until the potatoes become tender. Increase your oven temperature to 450 degrees F. Take out the foil, and cook for 8 minutes until potatoes become lightly browned.

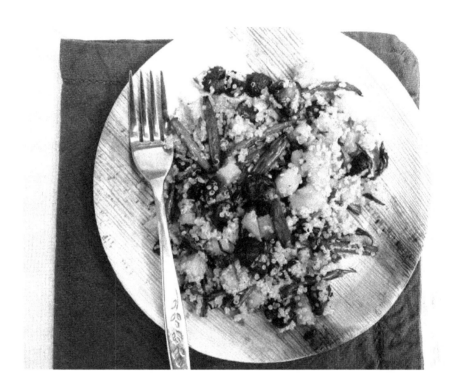

# Roasted Italian Kohlrabi and Asparagus

Ingredients

1 1/2 pounds kohlrabi, cut into chunks

2 tablespoons extra virgin olive oil

12 cloves garlic, thinly sliced

1 tsp. Italian seasoning

4 teaspoons dried thyme

2 teaspoons sea salt

1 bunch fresh asparagus, trimmed and cut into 1 inch pieces

Directions:

Preheat your oven to 425 degrees F. In a baking pan, combine the first 5 ingredients and 1/2 of the sea salt. Cover with foil. Bake 20 minutes in the oven. Combine the asparagus, oil, and salt. Cover, and cook for about 15 minutes, or until the kohlrabi becomes tender. Increase your oven temperature to 450 degrees F. Take out the foil, and cook for 8 minutes until kohlrabi become lightly browned.

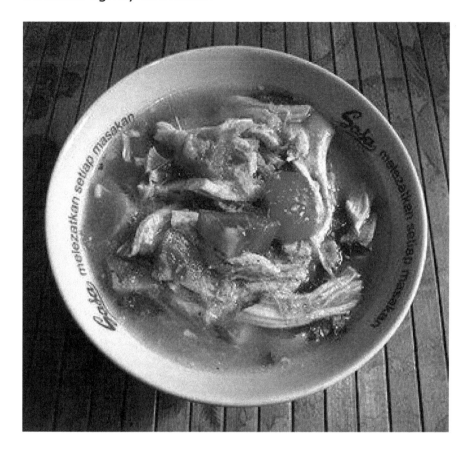

## Roasted Yucca Root, Turnips & Carrots

Ingredients

1/2 pound carrots, cut into chunks

½ pound yucca root, cut into chunks

½ pound turnips, cut into chunks

2 tablespoons extra virgin olive oil

12 cloves garlic, thinly sliced

1 tbsp. and 1 tsp. dried rosemary

4 teaspoons dried thyme

2 teaspoons sea salt

1 bunch fresh asparagus, trimmed and cut into 1 inch pieces

Directions:

Preheat your oven to 425 degrees F. In a baking pan, combine the first 7 ingredients and 1/2 of the sea salt. Cover with foil. Bake 20 minutes in the oven. Combine the asparagus, oil, and salt. Cover, and cook for about 15 minutes, or until the root vegetables become tender.

Increase your oven temperature to 450 degrees F. Take out the foil, and cook for 8 minutes until yucca root become lightly browned.

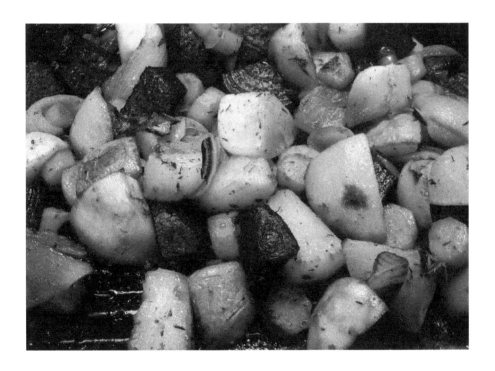

## Roasted Nutty Potato and Sweet Potato

Ingredients

1/2 pounds red potatoes, cut into chunks

½ pound sweet potatoes, cut into chunks

2 tablespoons peanut oil

12 cloves garlic, thinly sliced

1 tbsp. and 1 tsp. herbs de Provence

2 teaspoons sea salt

1 bunch fresh asparagus, trimmed and cut into 1 inch pieces

Directions:

Preheat your oven to 425 degrees F. In a baking pan, combine the first 6 ingredients and 1/2 of the sea salt. Cover with foil. Bake 20 minutes in the oven. Combine the asparagus, oil, and salt. Cover, and cook for about 15 minutes, or until the root vegetables become tender. Increase your oven temperature to 450 degrees F. Take out the foil, and cook for 8 minutes until potatoes become lightly browned.

## Roasted Yams and Asparagus

Ingredients

1/2 pound purple yam, cut into chunks

½ pound white yam, cut into chunks

½ pound sweet potato

 2 tablespoons canola olive oil

12 cloves garlic, thinly sliced

2 tsp. Italian seasoning

2 teaspoons sea salt

1 bunch fresh asparagus, trimmed and cut into 1 inch pieces


Directions:

Preheat your oven to 425 degrees F. In a baking pan, combine the first 6 ingredients and 1/2 of the sea salt. Cover with foil. Bake 20 minutes in the oven. Combine the asparagus, oil, and salt. Cover, and cook for about 15 minutes, or until the root vegetables become tender. Increase your oven temperature to 450 degrees F. Take out the foil, and cook for 8 minutes until potatoes become lightly browned.

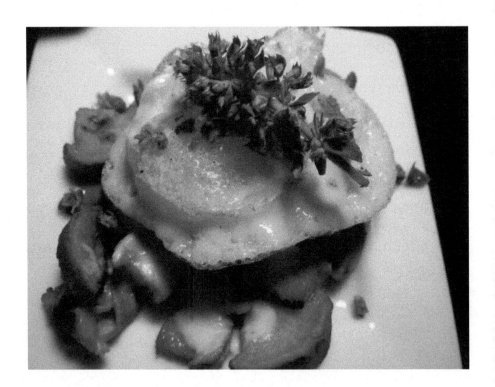

# Soups and Salads

## Zoodles Greek Salad
Prep Time 10 mins Cook Time 0 mins Servings: 4 -6

Ingredients

Juice of a lemon (about 1/4 cup)

1 Tablespoon balsamic vinegar

1 Tablespoon olive oil

1 teaspoon minced fresh oregano kosher salt & pepper

2 medium zucchini (peeled if desired)

1 cup grape or cherry tomatoes, halved

1/2 cup pitted kalamata olives, halved

2 oz. crumbled feta cheese (about 1/2 cup)

Instructions

In a small bowl, whisk together the lemon juice, balsamic vinegar, olive oil, oregano, and salt and pepper, to taste, and set the dressing aside.

Using, a vegetable spiral cutter, cut the zucchini into zucchini noodles.

In a large bowl, gently toss together the zucchini noodles, tomatoes, olives, feta and the dressing until combined and evenly coated.

Nutrition Info

Calories: 121kcal Carbohydrates: 6g Protein: 3g

Fat: 9g

Saturated Fat: 3g Cholesterol: 12mg Sodium: 433mg Potassium: 336mg Fiber: 2g

Sugar: 4g

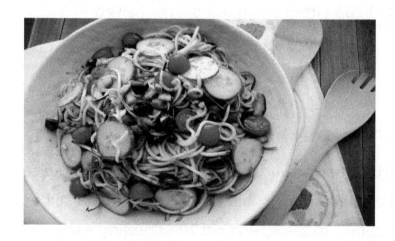

## Antipasto Cauliflower Salad

Servings: (8) 1/2 cup

Ingredients

2 cups of raw cauliflower, chopped

1/2 cup radicchio, chopped

1/2 cup artichoke hearts, chopped

1/3 cup fresh basil, chopped

1/2 cup freshly grated parmesan

3 Tbsp sundried tomatoes, chopped

3 Tbsp kalamata olives, chopped

1 clove garlic, minced

3 Tbsp balsamic vinegar

3 Tbsp extra virgin olive oil salt and pepper to taste

Instructions

First, cook your finely chopped cauliflower in the microwave for five minutes. Don't add any liquid or seasoning to it, just spread it on a microwave safe dish and zap it. Let the cauliflower cool while you prep the other ingredients.

Combine the radicchio, artichoke hearts, basil, parmesan, sundried tomatoes, olives, and garlic in a medium bowl.

In a smaller bowl, whisk together the olive oil and vinegar, then pour it over the salad. Toss to combine, and season with salt and pepper to taste. Can be served room temperature or chilled.

Nutrition Info

Calories: 102 Fat: 8g

Carbohydrates: 4g net Protein: 3g

# Charred Veggie and Fried Goat Cheese Salad

Servings 2

Ingredients

2 tablespoons poppy seeds

2 tablespoons sesame seeds 1 teaspoon onion flakes

1 teaspoon garlic flakes

4 ounces goat cheese, cut into

4 ½ in thick medallions

1      medium red bell pepper, seeds removed & cut into 8 pieces

½ cup baby portobello mushrooms, sliced

4 cups arugula, divided between two bowls

1 tablespoon avocado oil

Instructions

Combine the poppy and sesame seeds, onion, and garlic flakes in a small dish.

Coat each piece of goat cheese on both sides. Plate and place in the refrigerator until you are ready to fry the cheese. Prepare a skillet with nonstick spray and heat to medium. Char the peppers and mushrooms on both sides, just until the pieces begin to darken and the pepper softens. Add to the bowls of arugula.

Place the cold goat cheese in the skillet and fry on each side for about 30 seconds. This melts quickly so be gentle as you flip each piece!

Add the cheese to the salad and drizzle with avocado oil. Serve warm!

Nutrition Info

350 Calories

27.61 g Fat

7.08 g Net Carbs

16.09 g Protein.

## Simple Greek Salad

This Simple Greek Salad comes together in under five minutes. By using a few key flavors you can whip up a restaurant quality side in no time.

Prep Time: 10 minutes Total Time: 10 minutes
Servings: 6

Ingredients

1      cucumbers peeled and chopped

1 pint grape tomatoes halved

4 oz feta cheese cubed

2 tbsp fresh dill

2 tbsp extra virgin olive oil

Instructions

Combine the first four ingredients in a medium bowl. Drizzle with the olive oil. Toss lightly to combine.

Nutrition Info

Calories: 117 Carbohydrates: 6g Protein: 4g

Fat: 9g Saturated Fat: 4g Cholesterol: 17mg Sodium: 217mg Potassium: 335mg Fiber: 2g

Sugar: 4g

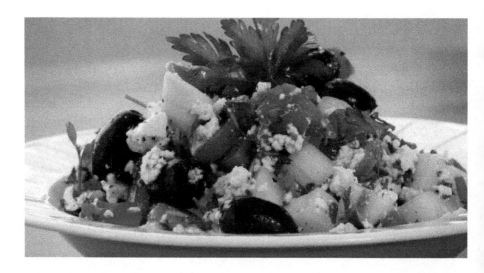

# Keto Asian Noodle Salad with Peanut Sauce

This easy vegetarian Keto Asian Noodle Salad can be made in advance for picnics, parties, or as meal prep for keto lunches all week! Low carb, Atkins, Paleo, gluten free, and can easily be made vegan

Prep Time: 10 minutes Total Time: 10 minutes Servings: 4 servings

Ingredients

For the salad:

1 cup shredded red cabbage

1 cup shredded green cabbage 1/4 cup chopped scallions

1/4 cup chopped cilantro

4 cups shiritake noodles (drained and rinsed) 1/4 cup chopped peanuts

For the dressing:

2 tablespoons minced ginger 1 teaspoon minced garlic

½ cup filtered water

1 tablespoon lime juice

1 tablespoon toasted sesame oil

1 tablespoon wheat-free soy sauce

1 tablespoon fish sauce (or coconut aminos for vegan)

¼ cup sugar free peanut butter

¼ teaspoon cayenne pepper

½ teaspoon kosher salt

1 tablespoon granulated erythritol sweetener

## Instructions

Combine all of the salad ingredients in a large bowl. Combine all of the dressing ingredients in a blender or magic bullet. Blend until smooth. Pour the dressing over the salad and toss to coat. Serve immediately, or store in an airtight container in the refrigerator for up to 5 days. Do not freeze.

## Nutrition Info

Serving Size: 1.5 cups Calories: 212 Fat: 16g Carbohydrates: 9g Fiber: 3g Protein: 7g

## Parsley Almond Pesto Barley Salad

(Prep time: 25 min| Cooking Time: 20 min | serve: 2)

Ingredients

½ cup water

¼ cup barley

1 cup broccoli florets

½ cup fresh parsley

1/8 cup almonds

1 tablespoon coconut oil

½ cup diced tomato

½ cup diced baby cucumber

¼ cup sliced celery

¼ cup crumbled goat cheese or more to taste

Salt to taste

Instructions

Pour the water into the Instant Pot and add the barley. Lock the lid into place. Select Pressure Cook or Manual, and adjust the pressure to High and the time to 15 minutes. Make sure the vent on top is set to Sealing. After cooking, naturally, release the pressure. Unlock and remove the lid. Drain the barley and let cool for about 5 minutes. Add parsley, almonds, and coconut oil together in a blender or food processor until the sauce is smooth.

Stir barley, broccoli, tomatoes, cucumbers, and celery together in a large bowl. Pour parsley sauce over barley mixture and toss to coat thoroughly. Sprinkle goat cheese over the top and season with salt.

Nutrition Facts

Calories 233, Total Fat 11.5g, Saturated Fat 6.8g, Cholesterol 2mg, Sodium 131mg, Total Carbohydrate

25.2g, Dietary Fiber 7.3g, Total Sugars 3.1g, Protein 7.2g

## Kale, Tomato, and Bulgur Salad

(Prep time: 15 min| Cooking Time: 0 min | serve: 2)

Ingredients

1 cup water

½ cup uncooked bulgur

½ cup fresh kale, chopped

2 hard-boiled eggs, chopped

1/8 cup walnuts, toasted

1/8 cup toasted sunflower seeds

1 tablespoon ranch dressing

Instructions

Pour the bulgur into the Instant Pot. Add the water and kosher salt. Lock the lid into place. Select Pressure Cook or Manual, and adjust the pressure to High and the time to 10 minutes. After cooking, let the pressure release naturally for 2 minutes, then quickly release any remaining pressure. Unlock the lid. Remove the pot from the base. Fluff the bulgur with a fork and let it cool for a few minutes. Transfer it to a medium bowl. Toss bulgur, kale, hard-boiled eggs, walnuts, and sunflower seeds in a large bowl until combined. Top with ranch dressing.

Nutrition Facts

Calories 272, Total Fat 11g, Saturated Fat 1.8g Cholesterol 164mg, Sodium 121mg, Total Carbohydrate 30.4g, Dietary Fiber 7.5g, Total Sugars 0.9g, Protein 12.9g

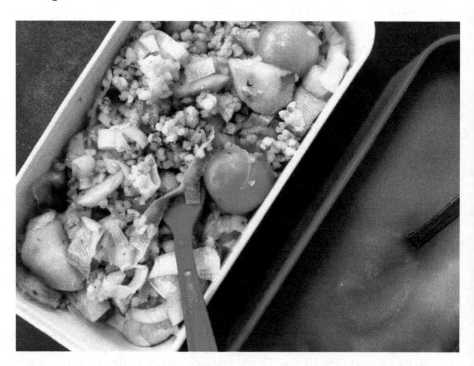

## Spinach, Amaranth, and Avocado Salad with Lemon Dijon Vinaigrette

(Prep time: 15 min| Cooking Time: 0 min | serve: 2)

Ingredients

½ cup amaranth

2 cups water

1 bunch spinach, torn into bite-sized pieces

¼ avocado, peeled, pitted, and diced

¼ cup chopped cucumbers

¼ cup chopped red bell peppers

1 tablespoon chopped red onions

½ tablespoon crumbled goat cheese

1/8 cup coconut oil

1 tablespoon lemon juice

½ tablespoon Dijon mustard

1/8 teaspoon sea salt

¼ teaspoon ground black pepper

## Instructions

Pour the amaranth into the Instant Pot. Add the water and kosher salt. Lock the lid into place. Select Pressure Cook or Manual, and adjust the pressure to High and the time to 10 minutes. After cooking, let the pressure release naturally for 2 minutes, then quickly release any remaining pressure. Unlock the lid. Remove the pot from the base add spinach. Top spinach with amaranth, avocado, cucumbers, bell peppers, red onions, and goat cheese. Whisk coconut oil, lemon juice, Dijon mustard, sea salt, and black pepper together in a bowl until the oil emulsifies into the dressing; pour over the salad.

## Nutrition Facts

Calories 460, Total Fat 25.2g, Saturated Fat 15.6g, Cholesterol 7mg, Sodium 342mg, Total

Carbohydrate 43.4g, Dietary Fiber 10.6g, Total Sugars 3.2g, Protein 15.1g

# Avocado, Pomegranate, and Buckwheat Salad

(Prep time: 15 min| Cooking Time: 15 min | serve: 2)

Ingredients

1 cup water

½ cup buckwheat

¼ avocado, peeled, pitted, and diced, or more to taste

¼ pomegranate, peeled and seeds separated, or more to taste

¼ tablespoon coconut oil

¼ tablespoon chopped fresh Parsley

½ lemon, juiced

¼ teaspoon kosher salt

Instructions

Pour the buckwheat into the Instant Pot. Add the water and kosher salt. Lock the lid into place. Select Pressure Cook or Manual, and adjust the pressure to High and the time to 10 minutes. After cooking, let the pressure release naturally for 2 minutes, then quickly release any remaining pressure. Unlock the lid. Transfer buckwheat to a large bowl and gently fold in avocado and pomegranate seeds. Drizzle coconut oil over buckwheat mixture and toss to coat; mix in parsley and lemon juice.

Nutrition Facts

Calories 243, Total Fat 8.2g, Saturated Fat 2.8g, Cholesterol 0mg, Sodium 6mg, Total Carbohydrate 35.9g, Dietary Fiber 6.7g, Total Sugars 2g, Protein 6.4g

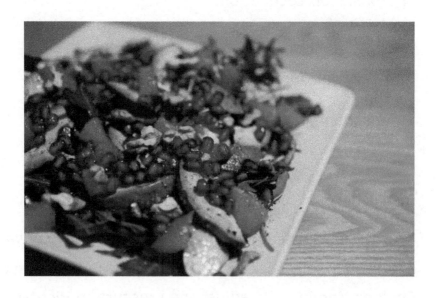

# Corn and Quinoa Salad with Lemon and Tahini

(Prep time: 10 min| Cooking Time: 10 min | serve: 2)

Ingredients

¼ cup sweet corn

¼ cup uncooked quinoa, rinsed

½ cup water

1 tablespoon chopped fresh parsley

1 small onion, chopped

½ teaspoon garlic powder

¼ tablespoon lemon juice

¼ tablespoon tahini

1 tablespoon coconut oil

Sea salt and ground black pepper to taste

Instructions

Pour the quinoa into the Instant Pot. Add the water and
kosher salt. Lock the lid into place. Select Pressure

Cook or Manual, and adjust the pressure to High and the time to 5 minutes. After cooking, let the pressure release naturally for 2 minutes, then quickly release any remaining pressure. Unlock the lid. Combine the sweet corn and quinoa in a mixing bowl with the parsley; set aside. In a separate bowl, whisk together the onions, garlic powder, lemon juice, tahini, and coconut oil. Season to taste with salt and pepper. Pour the dressing over the corn and quinoa mixture, and stir gently before serving.

Nutrition Facts

Calories 182, Total Fat 9.4g, Saturated Fat 6.2g, Cholesterol 0mg, Sodium 11mg, Total Carbohydrate

21.6g, Dietary Fiber 3.1g, Total Sugars 2.4g, Protein 4.5g

**Dinner**

**Tofu Teriyaki**

(Prep time: 15 min |Cooking Time: 30 min | serve: 2)

Ingredients

½ cup vegetable broth

1/8 cup tamari sauce

1/8 cup onion, peeled and chopped

½ tablespoon honey

½ tablespoon ginger powder

¼ tablespoon garlic powder

1 cup tofu, cubed

Instructions

Mix the broth, tamari, onion, honey, ginger powder, and garlic powder in an Instant Pot. Add the tofu, stir well, and lock the lid to the Instant Pot.

Press Pressure Cook on High Pressure for 10 minutes with the Keep Warm setting off.

When the machine has finished cooking, turn it off and let its pressure return to normal naturally, about 25 minutes. Unlatch the lid and open the cooker. Use tongs or a slotted spoon to transfer the tofu to a bowl.

Press the button for Sauté. Set it for High, More, or Custom 4000 F. Set the time for 15 minutes and press Start if necessary. Bring the sauce in the pot to a boil, stirring often. Continue boiling, stirring more frequently until almost constantly, until the sauce is a thick glaze for about 7 minutes. Turn off the Sauté function. Return the tofu and any juices to the cooker. Stir until the tofu is coated in the glaze. Transfer the pieces to a serving platter or plates.

Nutrition Facts

Calories 136, Total Fat 5.7g, Saturated Fat 1.2g, Cholesterol 0mg, Sodium 1213mg, Total Carbohydrate 10.1g, Dietary Fiber 1.7g, Total Sugars 6.2g, Protein 13.8g

## Zesty Lemon Jackfruit

(Prep time: 5 min |Cooking Time: 20 min | serve: 2)

Ingredients

½ teaspoon red chili powder

¼ teaspoon salt

¼ pepper

1 cup jackfruit

2 tablespoons coconut oil

1/2 small onion, chopped

1 teaspoon garlic powder

½ teaspoon dried basil, lightly crushed

1/8 cup lemon juice

Zest of one lemon

1 tablespoon chopped fresh coriander

Lemon slices for garnish

Basil, crushed

## Instructions

Mix red chili powder, salt, and pepper in a small bowl. Coat tops (Smooth side) of tofu in seasoning mixture.

Add coconut oil to the Instant Pot. Using the display panel, select the Sauté function. When oil gets hot, brown the jackfruit on both sides for about 3-4 minutes. Do not crowd the pot; you may have to work in batches. Transfer browned jackfruit to a shallow dish and cover loosely with foil. Add onion and remaining oil to the Instant Pot and sauté until soft, about 3- 4 minutes. Add garlic powder and crushed basil and cook for 1-2 minutes more. Add lemon juice and zest to the Instant Pot and deglaze by using a wooden spoon to scrape the brown bits from the bottom of the pot. Put the jackfruit back into the Instant Pot in one even layer, seasoned side up.

Turn the pot off by selecting Cancel, secure the lid, and make sure the vent is closed. Using the display panel, select the Manual or Pressure Cook function. Use the + /- keys and program the Instant Pot for 7 minutes.

When the time is up, let the pressure naturally release for 5 minutes, then quick-release the remaining pressure. Serve jackfruit topped with fresh coriander and lemon slices.

Nutrition Facts

Calories 207, Total Fat 13.9g, Saturated Fat 11.8g, Cholesterol 0mg, Sodium 295mg, Total Carbohydrate 23g, Dietary Fiber 2.2g, Total Sugars 1.1g, Protein 1.6g

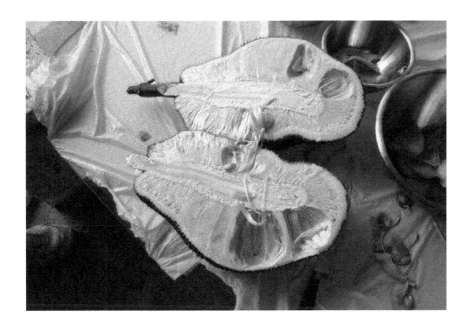

# Coconut Potato Curry

(Prep time: 5 min |Cooking Time: 10 min | serve: 2)

Ingredients Coconut Potato Curry:

½ tablespoon coconut oil

1 cup potatoes cubes

1 small onion, finely diced

1 teaspoon garlic powder

½ teaspoon ginger powder

1 cup coconut milk full fat

Spice Mixture:

½ tablespoon curry powder

½ tablespoon dried rosemary

½ teaspoon salt

¼ teaspoon chili powder

1/8 teaspoon pepper

¼ teaspoon cardamom

To Finish:

1tablespoon corn-starch

1/8 cup chopped cilantro for garnish

Instructions

Add coconut oil to the Instant Pot. Using the display panel select the Sauté function. When oil gets hot, brown the potatoes on both sides, 2-3 minutes per side. Add onion, garlic powder, and ginger powder to the pot and sauté 2 minutes. Stir in the Spice mixture Ingredients and cook for 1 minute more.

Add coconut milk to the Instant Pot and deglaze by using a wooden spoon to scrape the brown bits from the bottom of the pot. Turn the Instant Pot off by selecting Cancel, then secure the lid, making sure the vent is closed. Using the display panel, select the Manual or Pressure Cook function. Use the + /- keys and program the Instant Pot for 5 minutes.

When the time is up, quick-release the pressure.

Carefully remove 1/4 cup of the liquid from the Instant Pot and combine with the corn-starch. Stir into the Instant Pot until thickened. Serve with cilantro.

Nutrition Facts

Calories 431, Total Fat 32.6g, Saturated Fat 28.5g, Cholesterol 0mg, Sodium 615mg, Total Carbohydrate 28.3g, Dietary Fiber 5.8g, Total Sugars 6.5g, Protein 5.5g

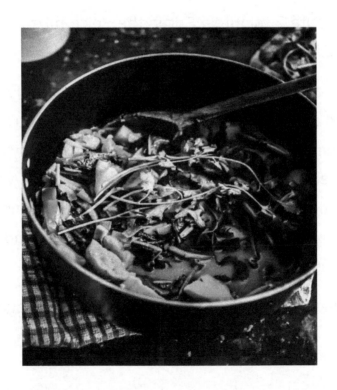

# Herb and Garlic Cottage Cheese

(Prep time: 35 min |Cooking Time: 20 min | serve: 2)

Ingredients

1 tablespoon coconut oil

½ tablespoon prepared Dijon mustard

½ tablespoon apple cider vinegar

1 teaspoon garlic powder

½ teaspoon pepper

¼ teaspoon salt

2 cups cottage cheese

1 tablespoon butter

1 teaspoon garlic powder

1/4 cup water

1/8 cup cream

½ tablespoon corn-starch

## Instructions

In a medium bowl, whisk together the marinade coconut oil, Dijon mustard, apple cider vinegar, garlic powder, pepper, salt. Add the cottage cheese and allow it to marinate for 30 minutes. Add coconut oil to the Instant Pot. Using the display panel select the Sauté function. When the coconut oil is melted, add garlic powder to the Instant Pot and sauté 2-3 minutes. Drain the cottage cheese, but reserve the marinade. Brown the cottage cheese on both sides, 3-4 minutes per side.

Add reserved marinade and 1/4 cup water to the pot and deglaze by using a wooden spoon to scrape the brown bits from the bottom of the pot. Put the cottage cheese back into the Instant Pot, turning once to coat. Turn the Instant Pot off by selecting Cancel, then secure the lid, making sure the vent is closed.

Using the display panel, select the Manual or Pressure Cook function. Use the + /- keys and program the Instant Pot for 5 minutes.

When the time is up, let the pressure naturally release for 10 minutes, then quick-release the remaining pressure. In a small bowl, mix cream and corn-starch. Stir into the Instant Pot until thickened, returning to

Sauté mode as needed. Serve cottage cheese topped with sauce.


Nutrition Facts

Calories 333, Total Fat 17.8g, Saturated Fat 12.8g, Cholesterol 36mg, Sodium 1346mg, Total Carbohydrate 10.1g, Dietary Fiber 0.3g, Total Sugars 1.4g, Protein 31.5g

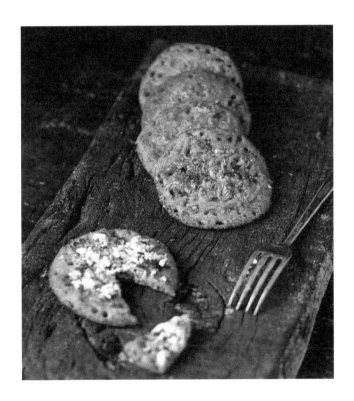

# Cilantro Lime Eggplant with Avocado

(Prep time: 5 min |Cooking Time: 20 min | serve: 2)

Ingredients

1 1/2 cups fresh sala

½ tablespoon taco seasoning

Zest and juice of 1 lime

¼ cup water

2 eggplants

1 jalapeno seeded and diced (optional)

½ cup chopped fresh cilantro

Avocado

Instructions

Add all ingredients to the Instant Pot and stir to combine. Secure the lid, making sure the vent is closed.

Using the display panel, select the Manual or Pressure Cook function. Use the + /- keys and program the Instant Pot for 12 minutes.

When the time is up, let the pressure naturally release for 10 minutes, then quick-release the remaining pressure.

Add cilantro. Stir to combine. Garnish with lime wedges and cheese.

Nutrition Facts

Calories 534, Total Fat 31.3g, Saturated Fat 7.5g, Cholesterol 23mg, Sodium 1049mg, Total Carbohydrate 56.9g, Dietary Fiber 28.2g, Total Sugars 18.6g, Protein 17.7g

# Southeast Asian Baked Turnip Greens & Carrots

Ingredients

½ pound turnips, peeled and cut into 1-inch chunks

½ pound carrots, peeled and cut into 1-inch chunks

½ pound parsnips, peeled and cut into 1-inch chunks

½ red onion, thinly sliced

½ cup vegetable broth

1 tbsp. extra virgin olive oil

½ tsp minced ginger

2 stalks lemon grass

8 cloves garlic, minced

Black pepper

½ pound fresh turnip greens, roughly chopped

Directions:

Put all of the ingredients in a slow cooker except the last one. Top with handfuls of turnip greens and stuff the slow cooker with it. If you can't fit it all in at once, let the first batch cook first and add some more turnip greens. Cook for 3or 4 hours on medium until turnips become soft. Scrape the sides and serve.

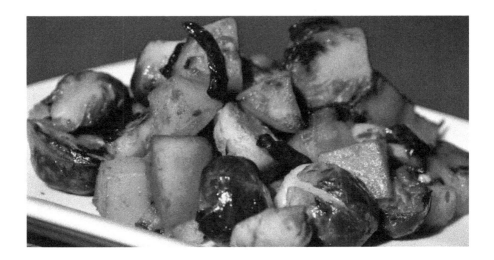

## Curried Watercress and Potatoes

Ingredients

1 ½ pounds potatoes, peeled and cut into 1-inch chunks

½ onion, thinly sliced

¼ cup water

½ vegetable stock cube, crumbled

1 tbsp. extra virgin olive oil

½ tsp cumin

½ tsp ground coriander

½ tsp garam masala

½ tsp hot chili powder

Black pepper

½ pound fresh Watercress, roughly chopped

Directions:

Put all of the ingredients in a slow cooker except the last one. Top with handfuls of watercress and stuff the slow cooker with it. If you can't fit it all in at once, let the first batch cook first and add some more watercress. Cook for 3or 4 hours on medium until potatoes become soft. Scrape the sides and serve.

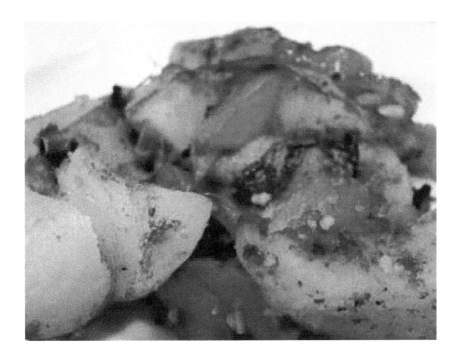

# Jalapeno Kale and Parsnips

Ingredients

1 ½ pounds parsnips, peeled and cut into

1-inch chunks

½ red onion, thinly sliced

¼ cup water

½ vegetable stock cube, crumbled

1 tbsp. extra virgin olive oil

½ tsp cumin

½ tsp jalapeno pepper, minced

1 ancho chili, minced Black pepper

½ pound Kale, roughly chopped

Directions:

Put all of the ingredients in a slow cooker except the last one. Top with handfuls of kale and stuff the slow cooker with it. If you can't fit it all in at once, let the first batch cook first and add some more Kale. Cook for

3or 4 hours on medium until parsnips become soft.
Scrape the sides and serve.

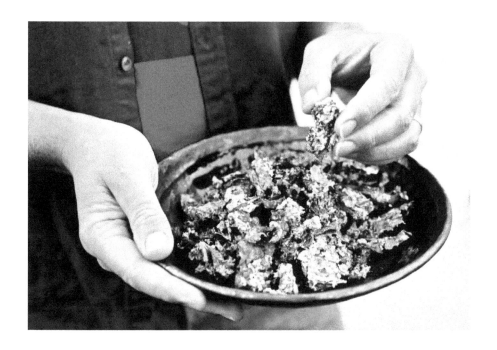

# Spinach and Zucchini Lasagna Recipe

Prep Time: 20 minutes Cook Time: 50 minutes

Total Time: 1 hour 10 minutes

Servings: 9 people

Ingredients

1 tablespoon extra virgin olive oil

½ onion - finely chopped 4 garlic cloves - crushed

1      tablespoons tomato paste

1 28-ounce can crushed tomatoes with the juice or 1¾ pounds of fresh tomatoes - peeled, seeded, and diced

Salt and ground fresh black pepper to taste 1 tablespoon fresh basil - chopped

3 cups spinach

15 ounces part-skim ricotta 1 large egg

½ cup freshly grated Parmesan cheese

4 medium zucchini - sliced ⅛-inch thick

16 ounces part-skim mozzarella cheese - shredded

½ teaspoon parsley - chopped

## Instructions

In a saucepan, heat the olive oil over medium heat.

Add the onions, and cook 4-5 minutes until they are soft and golden. Add the garlic, and sauté, being careful not to burn the garlic. Add the tomato paste and stir well. Add the chopped tomatoes, including the juice in case you are using canned tomatoes. Add salt and ground fresh black pepper. Bring to a low simmer, cover, and cook for 25-30 minutes. Finally, remove from the heat, and add the fresh basil and spinach. Stir well. Adjust the seasoning if necessary. Arrange the zucchini slices in a single layer on a baking sheet coated with cooking oil spray. Broil for 5-8 minutes. Remove from the oven. Wait about 5 minutes to remove any excess moisture with paper towels if necessary. (This part is very important to avoid the lasagna becoming too soupy.) Preheat the oven to 375°F.

In a medium bowl, mix the ricotta cheese, Parmesan cheese, and egg. Stir well.

In a 9x12-inch casserole, spread some tomato-spinach sauce on the bottom. Layer 5 or 6 zucchini slices to cover. Place some of the ricotta cheese mixture on the zucchini slices, and top with some mozzarella cheese. Repeat the layers until all your ingredients are used. Top with sauce and mozzarella. Cover the casserole dish with aluminum foil, and bake for 30 minutes. Uncover, and cook an additional 10-15 minutes. Let stand about 10 minutes before serving. Garnish with parsley.

Nutrition Info

Calories: 223kcal Carbohydrates: 10.6g Protein: 18.5g

Fat: 12.4g Cholesterol: 53mg Sugar: 4.4g

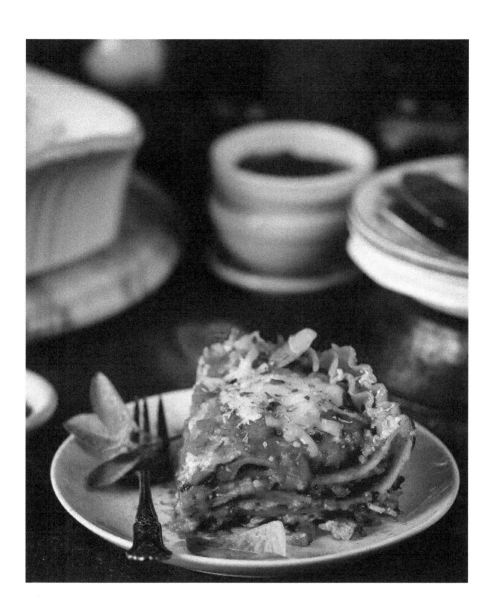

# Vegan Sesame Tofu and Eggplant

Servings 4

Ingredients

1 pound firm tofu, block

1 cup fresh cilantro, chopped, ~31g

3 tablespoons unseasoned rice vinegar 4 tablespoons toasted sesame oil

2 cloves garlic, finely minced

1 teaspoon crushed red pepper flakes 2 teaspoons Swerve confectioners

1      whole eggplant, ~458g 1 tablespoon olive oil Salt and pepper to taste

¼ cup sesame seeds

¼ cup soy sauce

Instructions

Preheat oven to 200°F. Remove the block of tofu from it's packaging and wrap with some paper towels. Place a plate on top of it and weigh it down. I used a really large tin of vegetables in this picture, but you can use anything handy. Let the tofu sit for a while to press some of the water out. Place about ¼ cup of cilantro, 3 tablespoons rice vinegar, 2 tablespoons toasted sesame oil, minced garlic, crushed red pepper flakes, and Swerve into a large mixing bowl. Whisk together. Peel and julienne the eggplant. You can julienne roughly by hand like I did, or use a mandolin with a julienne attachment for more precise "noodles." Mix the eggplant with the marinade. Add the tablespoon of olive oil to a skillet over medium-low heat. Cook the eggplant until it softens. The eggplant will soak up all of the liquids, so if you have issues with it sticking to the pan, feel free to add a little bit more sesame or olive oil. Just be sure to adjust your Nutrition Info tracking.

Turn the oven off. Stir the remaining cilantro into the eggplant then transfer the noodles to an oven safe dish. Cover with a lid, or foil, and place into the oven to keep warm. Wipe out the skillet and return to the stovetop to heat up again. Unwrap the tofu then cut into 8 slices. Spread the sesame seeds on a plate. Press both sides of each piece of tofu into the seeds. Add 2 tablespoons of sesame oil to the skillet. Fry both sides of the tofu for 5 minutes each, or until they start to crisp up. Pour the ¼ cup of soy sauce into the pan and coat the pieces of tofu. Cook until the tofu slices look browned and caramelized with the soy sauce.

Remove the noodles from the oven and plate the tofu on top.

Nutrition Info

292.75 Calories 24.45g Fats 6.87g Net Carbs 11.21g Protein.

**Sweets**

## No-bake keto cookies

No-bake keto cookies aka. keto almond clusters with 1.9 grams of net carbs per serving

Prep Time: 5 mins Total Time: 15 mins 10 cookies

Ingredients

1/3 cup almond butter

1 tablespoon Coconut oil

1/2 cup Sugar-free Chocolate Chips 1 1/4 cup Sliced almonds

1 tablespoon Chia seeds

Instructions

Cover a large plate or chopping board with a piece of parchment paper. Place the plate in the freezer while you prepare the cookie batter.

In a microwave-safe bowl, add almond butter, coconut oil, and sugar-free chocolate chips (or bars chopped in small pieces).

Microwave by 30 seconds burst, stirring between to avoid the almond butter to burn. It should take a maximum of 90 seconds to fully combine all your ingredients.

If you don't have a microwave, place all the ingredients into a small saucepan. Place under medium heat and stir all the time until chocolate melt and all the ingredients are combined.

Stir in the sliced almonds and chia seeds. You want to fully cover the almonds and seeds with the chocolate mixture.

Remove the plate from the freezer.

Spoon some cookie batter, then place the batter onto the prepared cold plate covered with parchment paper. As the plate is cold, the cookie shouldn't expand too much and the base should set fast. Leave 1 thumb space between each cookie just in case they expand slightly. Repeat until no more batter left.

You should be able to form 10 bite-size cookies.

Place the plate back in the freezer for 10 minutes or until the chocolate is firm and set.

Store your cookies in an airtight container in the fridge for up to 3 weeks. They are crunchier if stored in the fridge.

You can triple the recipe to meal prep your snack for the week and freeze those cookies in a zip bag for later. Defrost for 3-4 hours before eating.


Nutrition Info

Calories 141 Calories from Fat 113 Fat 12.5g19% Carbohydrates 4.9g2% Fiber 3g13% Sugar 0.9g1% Protein 4.5g

# Chocolate Avocado Cookies

Prep Time: 10 mins Cook Time: 12 mins Total Time: 22 mins 6 cookies

Ingredients

1 Avocado about 1/2 cup mashed avocado

1/4 cup Sugar-free flavored maple syrup or maple syrup (if not low carb)

1/2 cup Nut butter peanut butter or almond butter (if paleo) 1 Egg or chia egg if vegan

1/2 cup unsweetened cocoa powder 1/4 cup Sugar-free Chocolate Chips or choose your favorite one 1 teaspoon Vanilla extract 2-3 drops Monk Fruit Drops or Stevia Drops


Instructions

Preheat oven to 180°C (360°F)

Cover a baking sheet with parchment paper. Slightly oil the paper with 1/2 teaspoon of liquid vegetable oil (coconut or peanut oil). This will prevent the cookies to stick to the paper. Set aside.

In a food processor, with the S blade attachment, add ripe avocado and sugar-free maple syrup (or liquid sweetener you like). Process for 30 seconds until it forms a creamy avocado batter with no lumps.

Stop, add egg, nut butter, and cocoa powder. Process again for 30 seconds. Scrape down the bottom and side of the bowl and process for an extra 15 seconds to make sure all the batter is combined - no lumps.

Transfer the chocolate cookie batter onto a mixing bowl. It will bit moist and sticky that is what you want. Stir in chocolate chips and vanilla - if used.

Combine with a spatula until the chocolate chips are evenly incorporated. Test the batter and adjust with 2-3 drops of liquid stevia - only if you want a sweeter cookie. I did not add any to mine but if you have a sweet tooth I recommend few drops of stevia to make them sweeter. Add one drop at a time and see how it tastes.

Prepare a small bowl with warm water, dip a spoon in the water, and use that spoon to sample some chocolate cookie batter from your bowl. The water will prevent the batter to stick too much to your spoon.

Spoon the chocolate batter onto the baking sheet - I used another spoon to push the batter out of the first spoon. Use a silicone spoon or spatula to flatten the cookie into a cookie shape. The batter won't stick onto silicone which makes it easier to spread.

Repeat until you form 6 jumbo cookies. Those cookies won't spread so you don't need to leave more than half thumb space between each.

Sprinkle extra chocolate chips on top of each cookie if you like. Bake for 12-15 minutes or until the center is set.

Cool it down for 5 minutes on the baking sheet then transfer onto a cooling rack to cool down.

Store the cookies in the fridge for up to 5 days in an airtight container.

## Sweet Corn Muffins

Prep time: 10 min Cooking Time: 25 min serve: 2

Ingredients

½ cup coconut flour

1 tablespoon maple syrup

2 tablespoons cornmeal

¼ teaspoon baking powder

¼ teaspoon salt

1/8 cup sweet corn

1 egg, beaten

¼ cup applesauce

½ cup coconut milk

1 cup water

Instructions

Mix coconut flour, maple, cornmeal, baking powder, and salt in a large mixing bowl. Add sweet corn, egg, applesauce, and ¼ cup coconut milk to the flour mixture and beat with an electric hand mixer for 1 minute. Pour remaining milk into the batter and beat until just blended. Fill muffin tins 3/4 full of batter.

Pour 1 cup water into the Instant Pot. Place the trivet inside. Place the muffin cups on the rack or pan.

Secure the lid and set the Pressure Release valve to Sealing. Press the Pressure Cook or Manual button and set the cook time to 20 minutes.

When the Instant Pot beeps, allow the pressure to release naturally for 10 minutes, then carefully switch the Pressure Release valve to Venting. When fully released, open the lid. Carefully remove the muffins. Cool in the pans for 10 minutes before removing to cool completely on a wire rack.

Nutrition Facts

Calories 124, Total Fat 5.5g, Saturated Fat 3.9g, Cholesterol 41mg , Sodium 177mg, Total Carbohydrate

17.3g, Dietary Fiber 2.5g, Total Sugars 6.5g, Protein 3.6g

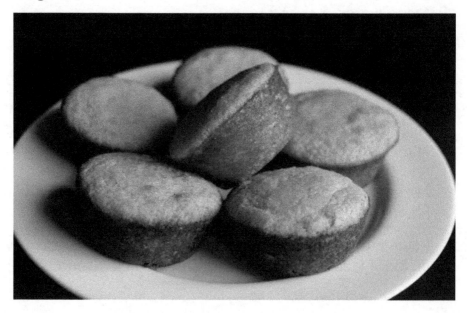

## Blueberry Pumpkin Muffins

Prep time: 15 min Cooking Time: 20 min serve: 2

Ingredients

½ cup coconut flour

1 tablespoon quick cooking oats

1 tablespoon honey

½ teaspoon baking powder

¼ teaspoon salt

½ teaspoon ground cinnamon

½ teaspoon nutmeg

¼ cup canned pumpkin

1/8 cup coconut milk

1 egg

1/8 cup butter, melted

¼ cup fresh blueberries

1 cup water


Instructions

Mix the coconut flour, oats, honey, baking powder, salt, cinnamon, and nutmeg in a mixing bowl until evenly blended. In a separate bowl, stir together the pumpkin, coconut milk, egg, and butter. Gradually stir in the flour mixture, just until all ingredients are moistened. Fold in the blueberries.

Pour 1 cup water into the Instant Pot. Place the trivet inside. Place the muffin cups on the rack or pan.

Secure the lid and set the Pressure Release valve to Sealing. Press the Pressure Cook or Manual button and set the cook time to 20 minutes.

When the Instant Pot beeps, allow the pressure to release naturally for 10 minutes, then carefully switch the Pressure Release valve to Venting. When fully released, open the lid. Carefully remove the muffins.

Nutrition Facts

Calories 125, Total Fat 9.1g, Saturated Fat 5.9g, Cholesterol 56mg , Sodium 210mg, Total Carbohydrate

9.9g, Dietary Fiber 1.8g , Total Sugars 6.3g, Protein 2.3g

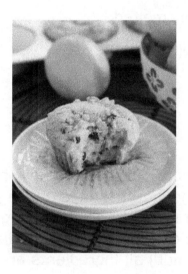

# Cornmeal Quinoa Poppy Seed Muffins

Prep time: 15 min Cooking Time: 20 min serve: 2
Ingredients

½ cup quinoa flour

½ cup coconut flour

½ tablespoon yellow cornmeal

¼ teaspoon poppy seeds

1 tablespoon maple syrup

¼ tablespoon grated lemon

¼ teaspoon baking powder

½ teaspoon baking soda

Pinch salt

¼ cup coconut milk

¼ tablespoon coconut oil

1 egg

¼ teaspoon vanilla extract

1 cup water

Instructions

Mix quinoa flour, coconut flour, cornmeal, poppy seeds, maple syrup, grated lemon, baking powder, baking soda, and salt in a bowl.

Whisk coconut milk, coconut oil, egg, and vanilla extract together in a separate bowl. Stir milk mixture into flour mixture until just combined. Pour batter into the prepared muffin cups.

Pour 1 cup water into the Instant Pot. Place the trivet inside. Place the muffin cups on the rack or pan.

Secure the lid and set the Pressure Release valve to Sealing. Press the Pressure Cook or Manual button and set the cook time to 20 minutes.

When the Instant Pot beeps, allow the pressure to release naturally for 10 minutes, then carefully switch the Pressure Release valve to Venting. When fully released, open the lid. Carefully remove the muffins.

Nutrition Facts

Calories 162, Total Fat 7.2g, Saturated Fat 4.7g, Cholesterol 41mg , Sodium 221mg, Total Carbohydrate 19.9g, Dietary Fiber 2.6g, Total Sugars 3.8g, Protein 5.1g

## Keto Egg Fast Snickerdoodle Crepes

A delicious keto egg fast crepe recipe based on the popular snickerdoodle cookie! Low carb, keto, lchf, egg fast, and Atkins diet friendly recipe.

Servings: Approximately 4 servings

Ingredients

For the crepes:

6 eggs

5 oz cream cheese, softened 1 tsp cinnamon

1 Tbsp granulated sugar substitute (Splenda, Swerve, Ideal, etc.)

butter for frying


For the filling:

8 Tbsp butter, softened

1/3 cup granulated sugar substitute 1 Tbsp (or more) cinnamon


Instructions

Blend all of the crepe ingredients (except the butter) together in a blender or magic bullet until smooth. Let the batter rest for 5 minutes.

Heat butter in a nonstick pan on medium heat until sizzling. Pour enough batter into the pan to form a 6 inch crepe. Cook for about 2 minutes, then flip and cook for an additional minute.

Remove and stack on a warm plate. You should end up with about 8 crepes.

Meanwhile, mix your sweetener and cinnamon in a small bowl or baggie until combined.

Stir half of the mixture into your softened butter until smooth. To serve, spread 1 Tbsp of the butter mixture onto the center of your crepe.

Roll up and sprinkle with about 1 tsp of additional sweetener/ cinnamon mixture.

Nutrition Info

Serving Size: 2 crepes, 2 Tbsp filling Calories: 434

Fat: 42g Carbohydrates: 2g net Protein: 12g

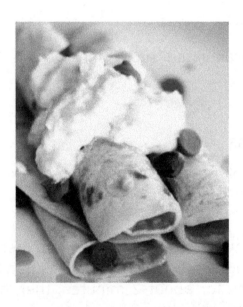

# Sun Dried Tomato Pesto Mug Cake

Servings 1 Sun Dried Tomato Pesto Mug Cake

Ingredients

Base

1 large egg

2 tablespoons butter

2 tablespoons almond flour

½ teaspoon baking powder

5 teaspoons sun dried tomato pesto 1 tablespoon almond flour

Pinch salt

Instructions

Get your mug ready! Add 1 Large Egg, 3 Tbsp. Honeyville Almond Flour, 2 Tbsp. of Room Temperature Butter, 5 tsp. Sun Dried Tomato Pesto, 1/2 tsp. Baking Powder and a pinch of salt.

Mix everything together well.

Microwave this for 75 seconds on high (power level 10).

Then, lightly slam your mug against a plate so that it comes out. Top with extra cheese sun dried tomato and a small wedge of fresh tomato!

# Keto Cannoli Stuffed Crepes

These Keto Cannoli Stuffed Crepes are perfect for any special occasion breakfast or brunch! Tastes like you're cheating, but they are low carb, gluten free, grain free, Atkins, and nut free too!

Prep Time: 15 minutes Cook Time: 20 minutes Total Time: 35 minutes Servings: 4 servings

Ingredients

For the crepes:

8 ounces cream cheese, softened

8 eggs

1/2 teaspoon ground cinnamon

1 tablespoon granulated erythritol sweetener 2 tablespoons butter, for the pan


For the cannoli filling:

6 ounces mascarpone cheese, softened 1 cup whole milk ricotta cheese

1/2 teaspoon lemon zest

1/2 teaspoon ground cinnamon

1/4 teaspoon unsweetened vanilla extract 1/4 cup powdered erythritol sweetener


For the optional chocolate drizzle (not included in Nutrition Info:)

3 squares of a Lindt 90% chocolate bar

Instructions

For the crepes:

Combine all of the crepes ingredients in a blender and blend until smooth.

Let the batter rest for 5 minutes and then give it a stir to break up any additional air bubbles.

Heat 1 teaspoon of butter in a 10 inch or larger nonstick saute pan over medium heat.

When the butter is melted and bubbling, pour in about 1/4 cup of batter (you can eyeball it) and if necessary, gently tilt the pan in a circular motion to create a 6-inch (-ish) round crepe.

Cook for two minutes, or until the top is no longer glossy and bubbles have formed almost to the middle of the crepe.

Carefully flip and cook for another 30 seconds. Remove and place on a plate.

Repeat until you have 8 usable crepes.

For the cannoli filling:

Place all of the filling ingredients in a medium-sized bowl and fold gently with a silicone spatula until fully combined.

Spoon the filling into a pastry bag fitted with a large star tube. (If you don't have a pastry bag, use a gallon sized plastic bag with the corner cut out to create a 1 inch wide opening.) Alternatively you can just smear it on the crepe with a spoon.

Pipe a line of filling down the center of one crepe.

Fold the right side over the filling, and then the left side over the top to create a roll.

Repeat with the remaining 7 crepes.

Serve immediately or store, covered, in the refrigerator for up to 3 days.

For the optional chocolate drizzle (not included in Nutrition Info):

Just before serving the crepes, place the squares of chocolate in a small bowl.

Microwave on high, uncovered, for 30 seconds. Stir. If not melted, microwave for another 10 seconds. Stir.

Scrape the melted chocolate into a small plastic bag and cut a tiny bit of one bottom corner off.

Gently squeeze the bag to drizzle the chocolate over the crepes.

Nutrition Info

Serving Size: 2 stuffed crepes Calories: 478 Fat: 42g Carbohydrates: 4g Fiber: 0g Protein: 16g

## Peanut Butter Granola Balls

Peanut Butter Granola Balls or Keto energy bites are healthy, no bake, vegan, peanut butter chia seeds and almonds balls with sugar free chocolate chips.

Prep Time: 10 mins Total Time: 20 mins

Servings: 12 granola balls

Ingredients

Dry ingredients

1 cup Sliced almonds 1/4 cup Pumpkin seeds 1 tablespoon Chia seeds

2 tablespoon Flaxseed meal

1/4 cup Unsweetened desiccated Coconut 1/4 teaspoon Salt

1/4 cup Sugar-free Chocolate Chips or dark chocolate chips

>85% cocoa or cocoa nibs Liquid ingredients

1/2 cup Natural Peanut butter smooth, unsalted

1/4 cup Sugar-free flavored maple syrup or liquid sweetener of choice

Chcoolate drizzle

1/4 cup Sugar-free Chocolate Chips 1/2 teaspoon Coconut oil

Instructions

In a large mixing bowl add all the dry ingredients, stir to combine, set aside. Note: you can add the chocolate chips now and they will melt in the next step giving a chocolate peanut butter flavor to the ball or you can choose to add the chocolate chips after step 3 to keep the crunchy chocolate chips bites in the balls.

In a small bowl, add the liquid ingredients: peanut butter and sugar-free liquid sweetener, microwave 45 seconds. This step will soften the peanut butter making it easier to combine with the dry ingredients. Don't over-warm.

Pour the liquid ingredients onto the dry ingredients, combine using a spatula until it forms a sticky batter that you can easily shape into granola balls. If you didn't add the chocolate chips in step 1, stir in now.

Slightly grease your hands with coconut oil, grab some dough and roll the granola balls. I recommend a 'golf ball' size to make 12 granola balls in total with this batter.

Roll the prepared granola balls in extra sliced almonds if you like to add some crunch on the sides. Place the granola ball on a plate that you have covered with parchment paper - this prevents the ball from sticking to the plate.

Repeat the rolling process until you form 12 granola balls. Place the plate in the freezer for 10 minutes to firm up the granola balls. Meanwhile melt the extra chocolate chips with coconut oil.

Remove the plate from the freezer, drizzle some melted chocolate on top of each granola ball. Place the plate in the freezer again for 5 minutes to set the chocolate drizzle.

Store up to 3 weeks in the fridge in an airtight container or up to 10 days in the pantry in a cookie jar.

Nutrition Info

Calories 145 Calories from Fat 107 Fat 11.9g Carbohydrates 7.5g Fiber 3.3g Sugar 1.5g Protein 5.3g

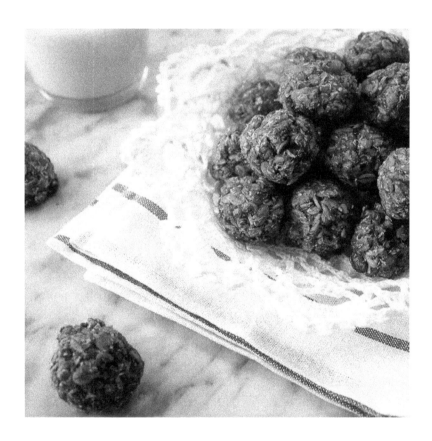

# Chocolate Peanut Butter Chia Seed Pudding

Ground chia seed pudding with Almond milk is a smooth chocolate peanut butter healthy dessert or breakfast.

Prep Time: 10 mins Total Time: 1 hr 10 mins

Servings: 6 pudding

Ingredients

2/3 cup Chia seeds whole, black or white or 1 cup ground chia seeds

3 tablespoons unsweetened cocoa powder

2 cups unsweetened Almond Breeze Almond Milk (or original if not keto)

2 tablespoons Natural Peanut butter

1/4 cup Sugar-free flavored maple syrup or any liquid sweetener you like (maple syrup, agave, brown rice syrup) 1/2 teaspoon Vanilla essence

1/4 teaspoon Salt


Instructions

Place the chia seed into a blender and blend for about 20 seconds to form ground chia seeds.

Add all the rest of the ingredients - order doesn't matter.

Blend again for 30 seconds to 1 minute until all the ingredients come together. If it sticks to the sides of the blender, you can stop the blender every 30 seconds, scrape down the side, and repeat until smooth. You can't over-process it!

Taste and adjust texture and sweetness. Add more almond milk, 1 tablespoon at a time for a runnier pudding. This may be useful if you replace the sugar-free liquid sweetener with crystal sweetener (erythritol or monk fruit sugar).

Transfer into ramekin or serving jar. Decorate with a dollop of fresh peanut butter, drizzle melted sugar-free dark chocolate and chopped peanuts.

Enjoy immediately or refrigerate for at least 1 hour for a fresher pudding.

Store for up to 4 days in the fridge in an airtight container.


Nutrition Info

Calories 203 Calories from Fat 111 Fat 12.3g19%

Carbohydrates 24.5g Fiber 19.6g82% Sugar 0.7g1% Protein 6.4g

Lightning Source UK Ltd.
Milton Keynes UK
UKHW021403070521
383306UK00005B/126